I0420166

Living a Healthy Lifestyle

Luis M. Rodriguez

Website: www.ahappybetterlife.com

Email: LMRod@ahappybetterlife.com

Disclaimer

The information provided in this book is designed to provide helpful information on the on the subjects discussed. This book is not meant to be used nor should it be used to diagnose or treat any medical condition. This book is not intended as a substitute for the medical advice of physicians. The reader should regularly consult a physician in matters relating to his/her health and particularly with respect to any symptoms that may require diagnosis or medical attention. Before beginning any new exercise program it is recommended that you seek medical advice from your personal physician.

The publisher and author are not responsible for any specific health or allergy needs that may require medical supervision and are not liable for any damages or negative consequences from any treatment, action, application or preparation to any person reading or following the information in this book.

Table of Contents

Introduction

Almost all of us want to have longer fuller lives so we can do more and spend more time with our family. But even though we want that, our style of living and our life choices say otherwise. Living a longer, loving more fulfilling life means living healthy. And living a healthy life doesn't only mean going to the gym and working out. It means we need to take care of our body and make easy to manage healthy choices in our day to day life.

We hear people talking or we read about living a healthy lifestyle, but how do we do it? A healthy person is somebody who doesn't smoke, is not over-weight, exercises and eats right. Sounds easy doesn't it? But how easy is it when we're trying to do it. In the process of attempting live a healthy life, it is important to take simple steps or make small manageable changes until we have totally incorporated healthy living into our lifestyle.

You only have one life so enjoy it to the fullest. Be happy, healthy and live longer!

Chapter 1

Introduction to a Healthy Lifestyle

How would you like to become a healthier and happy person just by making a few simple changes to your lifestyle? You'll have to make these changes to yourself in your entirety not just change the amount of exercise you do or change your diet. The secret to achieving a happier and a healthier you is to bring your body and mind into harmony. It is only when you are balanced in physically, mentally and spiritually that you can truly be healthy.

If you are healthy then you can be happier and can achieve success more easily in life. Here are just a few ways you can bring back harmony and balance to your life.

Exercise

This is an essential component that helps to tone your body, keep your heart and lungs healthy and detoxifies your system. Exercise can be anything from vigorous routines such as aerobics to simple walking. Choose your favorite activity and set aside a specific time of day and commit yourself to devoting a half-hour towards getting your body back into shape.

Eating Right

This is another essential step to maintaining a well-balanced life. Your body need the right amount of vitamins, nutrients and minerals to work at its best. Making changes to your diet is easy and can be accomplished by keeping away from fast foods which contain a lot of saturated fats and sugars and start including more whole grains, chicken, fish and plenty of green vegetables. Also, try eating fresh fruit instead of juice when available.

Supplements

Along with making changes to your diet you should include supplements such as vitamins, nutrients and minerals. Modern farming methods strip away many of the minerals contained in foods that your body require. Due to this you may be lacking in certain minerals and vitamins. By supplementing your diet with vitamin and mineral supplements, you can ensure you still get all the vital minerals, nutrients and vitamins you need in your daily diet.

Stress

Reducing the amount of stress you have in your life plays a vital part in how you are able to cope with life's little challenges. Stress can do much damage to your body and mind and has been linked with "burnout", fatigue, sleep problems, depression and it also weakens your immune system. Learning simple techniques on how to cope with stress and worry are essential to keeping yourself balanced and full of energy. There are a wide variety of techniques from simple breathing exercises, which can be done anywhere, to yoga, which is a full system for relaxation and de-stressing, to meditation. There are many books, DVDS and CDS available on the subject which you can use at home or there are classes you can attend.

Have Fun

Lastly but by no means the least important is keeping life fun, doing something you enjoy doing which will make you feel relaxed and happy each day. No you are not being selfish by taking time out each day just for yourself, this time is essential. It is just as important as exercising, eating right and reducing stress. Your time could be spent doing a hobby or pastime that you enjoy, sitting quietly and reading, taking a hot bubble bath while listening to your favorite music or spending quality time with your family or friends.   It can be anything as long as it's something you like and enjoying doing.

12 Ways to Improve your Health

The biggest step to achieving better health is admitting that you need to make changes towards becoming healthier and fitter. Here are a few ways to help you improve your health and become a new and improved you.

Make it a goal to obtain a healthier outlook on life which will undoubtedly lead to a healthier you. If you are determined to attain a better state of health, making it a reality will be all even easier.

Support your new way of thinking by learning everything you can about different ways of achieving better health and living a healthier lifestyle. You can use the internet, books, DVDS, clubs, gyms and support groups to your benefit. Finding out as much as you can about living a healthy lifestyle gives you a great base to work from.

You have to start somewhere so start by taking a look at your kitchen and reorganizing in preparation for your new way of life. Reorganize your kitchen cabinets, cupboards and refrigerator to ensure that there are no signs of the old you and replace them with the things that will help you in your new lifestyle.

Replace old food with healthier choices and don't forget to purchase any small appliances which you will need to support your healthier way of eating such as blenders and food scales.

Get a large planning calendar, pin it up in your kitchen and mark the day when you choose to begin your new lifestyle and stick to it no matter what.

From day one keep a journal. This can either be a traditional one or you can use your computer. You should include all thoughts and feelings about your new lifestyle along with all the changes you see about yourself. This is essential so that you can look back and see the improvement that's occurring due to your positive outlook and the changes you have made.

Positive thoughts and self-talk or affirmations are a necessity. They will give you confidence as you're starting out and will continue to take you through the tough times which will often occur early in the process.

Along with changes to your diet you will also have to make changes in the amount of exercise you do per day. While good healthy food is essential, exercise is just as important to help ward off the onset of diseases such as heart disease as well as helping you to firm up your body or lose those few pounds that just won't go away.

Give up any bad habits such as smoking or drinking. You will never reach your optimal peak state of health while you are puffing away on cigarettes or drinking on a regular basis.

Make sure that you get the recommended portions of fruit and vegetables per day on your new regimen. Fruit and vegetables are packed full of essential vitamins and nutrients.

Make sure you learn ways to eliminate as much stress from your life as you possibly can. There are many ways to do this with at least one of them sure to be suitable for your situation.

Cut out excess salt, sugar and fatty foods from your diet. This will effectively lower your cholesterol and blood pressure.

Where to Find Information on Nutrition

The best place to find out all you need to know about nutrition is on the United States Department of Agriculture (USDA) website. The USDA offers recommendations about what they find to be healthy eating-related habits for the general public. Their information covers these main areas of focus: nutrition pyramid, needed nutrients, weight management, physical fitness and food safety.

There is also a food pyramid on their website which has revised dietary guidelines and it is color coded to help you decide which foods to eat in order to maintain a healthy lifestyle.

Chapter 2

Look Your Best and Feel Even Better

How you look on the outside very often reflects how you are feeling on the inside. If you know you look good on the outside and are getting praise and compliments this automatically gives you a boost and makes you feel good. Some of the ways to looking better on the outside and ultimately feeling better include eating a well-balanced diet, exercising, and taking general care of your body and also your state of mental health.

Be Active

Daily exercise not only helps you to lose those few extra pounds but also tones your muscles leaving you looking and feeling better. Another benefit is it keeps you healthy which strengthens your immune system thereby making it easier to ward off disease and illness. There are many forms of exercise and it doesn't have to be expensive. You can buy inexpensive or used basic gym equipment to use in your own home or even take up a form of exercise which doesn't cost a penny, for example walking. In order to maintain the peak of health you should aim to exercise for at least 30 minutes per day every day of the week while maintaining a healthy balanced diet.

Balancing Your Meals

A well balanced diet is one that includes bread, cereals, fish, lean meats, chicken, potatoes, dairy products and plenty of fresh fruits and vegetables which are rich in vitamins and minerals. If you are trying to lose a few pounds then it is essential that you don't eat more calories per day than you are burning off. Cutting down on foods rich in salt, fats and carbohydrates is essential to maintaining a healthy body and along with exercise not only makes you look better but can help to counteract the onset of many health related problems.

The Importance of Being Mentally Healthy

Your mental health, your feelings and thoughts can also make a huge difference as to how you feel on the outside and inside. If you have negative thoughts and feelings running through your mind then your whole outlook will be one of negativity that leads to low self-confidence and low self-image. Meditation and daily affirmations can help you to change your pattern of thinking and increase your self-confidence.

All of the above when combined together can lead to a healthier and happier person who not only looks good on the outside and oozes self-confidence, but is also healthier and fitter on the inside with a better outlook on life and the ability to cope with life's little challenges.

Maintaining Your Proper Weight

Being overweight not only looks unsightly and makes you feel less attractive it also poses a far greater risk, a risk to your health. Being overweight has been linked to many conditions affecting not only your physical health but also your mental health.

Studies have shown that people who are overweight and don't exercise regularly are more at risk of being depressed than those who exercise on a regular basis and eat a well-balanced diet. Experts also agree that the more overweight a person is the more likely they are to suffer severe health problems. However once a person takes steps to start losing weight and changing their lifestyle, then the percentage starts to drop.

If you are overweight even just losing 10 or 20 pounds will help you reduce the increased associated risks to your health. You should definitely consider losing weight if you are overweight and if any of the following conditions apply to you.

If there is a history in your family of certain chronic diseases such as heart conditions or diabetes you could be at risk to develop these conditions if you are overweight.

If there are any pre-existing medical conditions such as high blood pressure, high cholesterol and high levels of sugar which are all signs of illness due to being overweight.

Is your body apple shaped? That is do you carry more weight around your stomach? If so then you are at a higher risk of developing diabetes, some forms of cancer or developing heart problems.

Health Dangers Associated with Being Overweight

Problems with the gallbladder and especially gallstones

High blood pressure

Developing certain types of cancer

Developing diabetes

Developing gout

Developing problems with your breathing such as sleep apnea, which causes a person to pause when breathing while asleep

Chest problems such as asthma or bronchitis

Gallbladder Problems

Although it is not clear why, being overweight can have an effect on the gallbladder, gallstones are a very common problem in someone who is overweight and causes severe problems with those who are obese.

9

Heart Disease

Being overweight makes you twice as likely to suffer from high blood pressure which is a major cause of strokes and a big risk factor in heart disease. Being overweight can lead to a condition known as angina. Angina is a pain felt in the chest caused by a decrease in oxygen to the heart. Being severely overweight or obese has been known to cause sudden death without any of the warning signs of a stroke.

Diabetes

Being overweight has been linked to type 2 diabetes and is a known contributor to heart disease and blindness. People who are overweight are twice as likely to suffer from type 2 diabetes as those who are of normal weight.

Your Cholesterol Levels

Monitoring your cholesterol and maintaining a healthy level is essential if you want to remain healthy. There are many ways you can reduce your cholesterol to ensure it remains at healthy levels and avoid illnesses such as heart disease.

Changing your diet and eating habits is by far one of the easiest ways of lowering your cholesterol and can be accomplished in some of the following ways:

Burn off at least as many calories as you eat during the course of a day

Make sure that you get at least 30 minutes of exercise every day of the week

Eat a wide variety of foods that are rich in nutrients

Include at least 5 portions of fruit and vegetables per day

Eat lots of high-fiber, wholegrain foods

Include fish in your diet at least twice a week

Cut out foods poor in nutrients

Cut down on the amount of trans-fat and saturated fat foods

In order to reduce trans-fat in your diet cut out foods containing partially hydrogenated vegetable oil

Remove the skin from chicken and eat only lean meat

Only include fat free and low fat dairy products

Include very little or no salt in your food

Drink alcohol in moderation

Always read the nutritional labels on food

You can also keep your cholesterol under control by exercising on a regular basis. Here are a just a few tips for getting started on a fitness program:

Start off slowly and gradually build up until you are getting 30 minutes of exercise per day

Make your daily workout a part of your life by doing it at the same time every day whenever possible

Make sure you drink enough water to ensure that you don't dehydrate

Enjoy your workout by joining a gym or working out with a friend

Keep a journal of your workout and write down the benefits you feel after exercising

Walk instead of taking the elevator, leave the car at home or walk or cycle to work

Vary your routine, go swimming one day, cycling the next, walking etc...

If you don't feel well, take a break from exercising and pick back up when you are feeling better

Make changes to your lifestyle that are both beneficial and helpful in lowering your cholesterol such as:

Getting nutritional and physical advice from a healthcare professional

Always read food labels so you know how much fat, sodium and other ingredients you are eating in your diet

If you smoke or drink then seriously consider giving it up

Can Diet Programs Really Work

There are many diet programs on the market today and many of you who have struggled with the need to lose a few pounds may have even tried a few of them. Some of you may have had some success while others failed miserably. Keep in mind that these programs are not magic and just like any other form of dieting the success behind it is all is on your shoulders and not the plan to lose weight. Sadly there is no magic formula which will help you to shed the pounds overnight while you sleep. Understanding why any diet does not work is critical for success and diet programs are no exception. So why do so many of us fail when it comes to dieting?

Sticking with the Plan

The biggest mistake that many of us make is not sticking to the plan. Diet programs normally require you to pay a membership fee which obligates you and gives you the commitment needed to follow through. These programs depend on you to keep track of what you eat and to take full advantage of the support that the program provides. The diets in these programs rely on counting calories or points with values assigned to the foods you eat. Points are assigned to each food based on the amount of calories and fat content within that particular food. You are allowed a certain number of points throughout the day based on your sex and weight. The system will work if the number of points per day are not exceeded but if you continually exceed the recommended daily allotted amount of points then quite simply you are not going to lose weight and indeed you could in fact gain weight.

Keeping Track of Your Progress

For any diet program to be successful it is essential that you keep some kind of log or journal in order to track of the foods you eat throughout the day. Relying on your memory to keep up with everything you eat is not the best way to do this.

Getting Rid of Those Unwanted Pounds

Sometimes you just want to kick start an exercise program or lose some weight in order to look good for an upcoming event or you just want to feel better and fit into your clothes comfortably. For those and any other occasions where it would be nice to lose a few pounds quickly, here are a few ways to help you achieve just that.

Make Time Not Excuses

Don't make any excuses! Your health and fitness is a priority and there is no better time than now to begin to shed that weight. If you don't set aside time and schedule fitness goals as part of your regular daily routine, then you are not planning to succeed but rather failing to plan. So grab your day planner and schedule at least 30 minutes a day for working out with some type of physical fitness activity.

Plan Your Attack

Next do a little homework and plan your attack on those extra pounds. You can choose among many popular fitness and weight loss plans like Weight Watchers, the Suzanne Somers Weight Loss Program, the Mayo Clinic Plan, Atkins, Bill Philips Body for Life Program, Jenny Craig, Slim-Fast and more. Or you can head out to your local gym and hire a trainer or just get moving on your own keeping track of the number of repetitions and resistance you're doing.

Keep a Positive Attitude

Make an attitude adjustment so that you have a positive and healthy outlook for accomplishing your fitness goals. For help getting this mindset and keeping it going throughout your program, head to your local library for motivational and inspirational books, audio cassettes, DVDs, videos and articles. Also look on the Internet for these helpful tools: articles, MP3 and other audio files, videos, e-books, reports and training examples.

Adjust Your Eating Habits

Take charge of your nutritional needs by setting up a good diet or choosing a good diet plan. A good place to look is online where many popular diet plans can be easily found. Some even offer a community forum for reaching out to new healthy friends online, meal planning and journaling and lots more. You can also head out to your local library for other helpful materials.

Keep Track of Your Journey

Grab a notebook and journey your way to your goals and beyond. Clearly write out what you want to accomplish, by what date and how you intend to get there using which methods. For example: working out 30 minutes a day and eating right following the Weight Watchers program guidelines.

Be Realistic

Be realistic when setting your weight loss goals and focus on what works best for you. Losing too much weight too quickly often results in the weight returning.

Share Your Weight Loss Plan to Encourage Others

If you have been successful at devising and sticking to a weight loss plan then why not share your plan and success with others who are striving to have the same success as you. There is nothing like encouragement to motivate others to see a plan through to success. And if they see someone else who is successful they are more likely to stick with a plan and achieve similar success in their life. Sharing and motivating each other is the number one reason why weight loss clubs, such as weight watchers, have such a high success rate. Knowing you are not the only one out there who is struggling and needs to shed a few pounds can make a huge difference. So if you have been successful with your weight loss plan then why not provide some inspiration and share it with others. A few of the many ways you can do this is by:

Blogging

Writing a blog allows you to get your thoughts and ideas out there to millions of people throughout the world. There are many websites that now offer free blog space and this can be ideal for getting your story out to the world. A blog is kind of an online diary which is your space to share your thoughts, feelings and ideas. Use your blog to share your successful weight loss plan and write down all that it took to get you where you are today. You can include the plan you used along with exercise routines and menus that you followed. Include your thoughts and feelings as you went through your journey to encourage people and show them that anything is possible.

Meet Up Groups

If you have a group of friends who are wanting to diet, then get together weekly or as often as you want to provide support for each other. Get together once a week for example and weigh yourselves for accountability and motivation. Share how you did the preceding week and encourage those who may have had some setbacks. Keep written records for all members of the group and plot your progress weekly. If one of you has been particularly successful in the past with your weight loss plan then maybe you are the one to lead the group and encourage other members to follow a similar plan.

Consider Turning Your Success into a Book

If you have had great success on your weight loss plan then consider writing a short e-book about your experiences and success in order to encourage others. It doesn't have to be anything fancy just something to show others your journey to weight lost success. It's a great, fun way to get your success story out there and to give others the motivation and encouragement they might need.

Chapter 3

Active Body Healthy Body

Stay Healthy by Simply Walking

Walking is the best form of exercise you can do to achieve better health and a fitter you and it doesn't cost anything. Anyone regardless of age can begin a sensibly walking regimen and it's something you can do alone or with friends.

When first starting out be sure to not overdo it, maybe no more that 10 to 15 minutes per day if you haven't been active at all. There are many ways you can fit this into your daily routine without too much trouble. Just consider when and where you could alter your routine and walk instead of taking the car or bus.

The benefits of walking are numerous and beneficial for your health and well-being and by simply altering your routine and walking daily you will:

See an increase in your overall fitness and the firmness of your muscles

Feel good and look better

Find that your energy level increases

Feel less stressed

Find that your sleep pattern changes and you'll sleep better and feel more rested

Begin to reduce the risk of heart disease

Reduce the risk of developing certain types of cancer

Find that you won't get depressed as easily as you once did

Your outlook on life in general and the way you deal with things changes for the better

You lose weight and look better

You find that your muscles, joints and bones are stronger

You reduce the risk of developing diabetes

You can start gaining all these benefits and more simply by increasing the amount of walking you do daily and by just being more active. In order to get the optimum health and fitness from walking you should strive to walk at a moderate pace. A moderate pace means walking faster than you normally do but not so fast that you're over exerting yourself. A good rule of thumb is being able to hold a conversation without getting breathless.

Not only will you feel better and look better once you have been on your new regimen for a while but you will feel many more benefits health wise and be well on the way to leading a more productive, happier and healthier lifestyle.

Benefits of Running

Running isn't just for runners anymore. Running just three days a week for 30 minutes has been proven to help maintain healthy weight as well as improve attitude and motivation. In short, running can help you become happier, healthier and stress free. Here's how:

Better Health

Running is not just an athlete's sport. Although you probably won't win he Boston Marathon, running can be a very healthy activity whether you choose to compete in races or not. In order to achieve optimal health benefits from running you should work yourself up to a level of being able to run at least 30 minutes at a time three or four days a week.

The best part about running is that you can do it anywhere. You'll probably need to invest in a good pair of running shoes so as not to injure yourself. Consider going to your local running store and have them fit you with the right type of shoes. The key here is not to have the cheapest shoes, the most expensive shoes or the nicest looking shoes, but to have the right shoes for your feet.

Better Attitude

Running, more than many other sports, can help develop a happier and healthier attitude towards life. If you can motivate yourself to get out there to run three days a week you will definitely begin to notice a difference. Most people find that after they have been running for a few weeks that it becomes addicting in an enjoyable way. The lessons you learn from running will help you become a more positive person and will teach you that anything is possible if you put your mind to it.

If you run with a negative attitude however, you'll find that you won't get very far or you will eventually just give up altogether. In order to motivate yourself to keep on running remember why you are doing it. You want better health, a better body and pride in knowing that you can do this. Amazing things start to happen when you keep your reasons in front of you. You will see the change from the old you to a new and healthier you. After a while running will become so enjoyable that you will look forward to your daily run.

Once you reach this level, you will find yourself with a more positive attitude. Running is one of the best attitude adjusters there is and once you start to look forward to running, you'll find yourself thinking positively about all aspects of your life.

Motivation

After you conquer the first 30 minutes of non-stop running, you will probably find yourself wondering if you could run further or faster. You can test this by finding a 5k or 10k race within driving distance. There are 5K runs almost every weekend and this can help you gauge how fast you can run. These races can serve as a great motivator for you and your newfound hobby. Run your first one without regard for time, just finish. After that, you will probably find yourself looking to improve your personal run time.

Ride Your Way to Better Health

To gain benefits from cycling you don't have to be super fit or an athlete. The benefits of bicycling are great and it is a fun way to get that much needed exercise.

Bicycling to Lose Weight

If you are trying to shed a few pounds, dieting alone isn't as effective as combining it with some type of regular exercise. If you cycle on a daily basis then it will not only help you burn a large number of calories during your workout but it will also raise your metabolism and help you burn even more calories throughout the day. Bicycling along a flat road or path at 12 mph will help you to burn off roughly 450 calories an hour. And even when you stop, your metabolism is still speeding ahead continuing to burn calories.

Not only can bicycling help you to lose weight and keep it off, it is also provides other health benefits. By cycling at least 20 miles per week you can help to reduce your risk of developing heart disease by half compared to those who don't do anything at all.

Bicycling's Other Benefits

Bicycling is considered an aerobic form of exercise meaning that this type of exercise is particularly beneficial to the lungs and heart. Your lungs expand with the effort of pedaling which allows you to get more oxygen into your body. This in turn makes your heart beat faster which sends the oxygen throughout your body. Developing powerful lungs and a strong heart will definitely put you on the road to improved overall fitness.

Just by bicycling a few miles per day you will begin to feel fitter, healthier and you will find yourself in much better shape. You will notice your muscles begin to firm up. Your thighs, backside and calf muscles will gain the biggest benefit from bicycling as these are the muscles that you will use the most. Soon you will notice that you no longer get winded walking up a flight of stairs. However the best part is that the more you bicycle the more you will enjoy it and you'll begin to look forward to your next outing.

Bicycling can also be beneficial when you are feeling down or if you suffer from stress, anxiety or depression. Exercise releases endorphins into our bloodstream and these endorphins bring about a feeling of happiness and contentment which is a great way to combat stress and depression.

Bicycling can be done almost anywhere you live and it doesn't have to be expensive. It is a relatively safe sport and when you follow a few simple guidelines it can also be enjoyed as a family adventure.

Here are a few simple tips to help you get the most out of bicycling

>Always carry a puncture repair kit

>Make sure you take a water bottle with you especially on long rides in the countryside

Keep your tires inflated to the required level to make your ride go smoother and easier

For safety always make sure you wear a bicycle helmet

Always have lights and reflectors on your bicycle to make sure you are seen

When bicycling at night, be sure to wear bright colors or preferably some sort of reflective material

Yoga and Your Body Weight

Many people are first drawn to yoga as a way to keep their bodies fit and supple while others come seeking relief for a specific ailment like tension or backache. Whatever your reason, yoga can be a tool used in giving you what you came for and more.

Though the practice of yoga is closely associated to ancient texts, beliefs and values, it also yields benefits useful for today's busy lives. Here are just some of the reasons more and more people are beginning to practice yoga:

Yoga relaxes the body and the mind. Even in the midst of stressful environments, yoga helps control breathing and clears the mind of cluttered thoughts leaving only deep physical and mental refreshment.

Yoga can help normalize body weight. For people who are either overweight or underweight, yoga exercises can help you achieve your desired weight. The principles of balance and moderation in physical activity and diet under yoga can also lead to a healthier lifestyle.

Yoga improves your resistance to disease. The postures and movements in yoga massage the internal organs enhancing blood circulation and functionality thus decreasing the risk of illness.

Yoga increasing your energy level and productivity. In as little as 20 minutes, yoga can replenish the mind and body with precious energy needed to keep up with daily tasks and challenges.

Yoga leads to genuine inner contentment and self-actualization. Meditation, one of the aspects of yoga, focuses the mind while taking it away from the distractions of your busy world and leading it to a place of genuine peace and happiness.

Yoga is a method of learning that aims to unite the mind, body and spirit through these three main yoga structures: Exercise, Breathing, and Meditation. The exercises of yoga are designed to gently place pressure on the glandular systems of the body thereby Increasing its efficiency and providing your body with total health.

The body is looked upon as the primary instrument that enables us to work and evolve in the world. A yoga student therefore treats it with great care and respect. The breathing techniques are based on the belief that breath is the source of life in the body. Yoga students gently increase their breath control to improve the health and the function of both body and mind. These two systems prepare the body and mind for meditation making it easier for students to achieve a quiet mind and be free from life's everyday stress.

Regular practice of yoga produces a clear, bright mind and a strong, capable body.

Chapter 4

Identifying Different Illnesses

Chronic Illness

There are many challenges you may face when dealing with chronic illness. If you have been diagnosed with having a long lasting health condition, then understanding it and learning what you can do to manage it can go a long way in helping you overcome it.

Having a chronic illness doesn't necessarily mean that it is dangerous or deadly. Asthma, diabetes and arthritis are all classified as chronic conditions and these can be kept under control with medication and supervision. Provided you take care of yourself and have the proper treatment, even with these conditions you can lead a normal and healthy life. Although the underlying condition won't go away and is always there, it can be controlled successfully.

Many people who have conditions such as asthma for example don't consider themselves as having a chronic condition because they feel relatively well most of the time. However there are others who are affected not only physically but also emotionally, socially and for some even financially. The severity in which it affects you is determined by the severity of your condition and the treatment involved in your particular situation. Whichever way you are affected it may sometimes take time to accept and adjust to your condition.

There is a certain process that you will go through whatever your illness, this is known as the coping process. When first diagnosed with chronic illness you may have many different feelings such as anger, worry, confusion and vulnerability; these being the most common.

The next stage is wanting to know and learn everything you can about your illness. This is a normal reaction because by gaining insight and knowledge into the condition, it makes it less frightening and you can feel more in control.

The third stage is developing confidence in the treatment you have been given for your condition. Begin by accepting that the medication or treatment you've being given will help to relieve symptoms and attacks and give you a sense of normalcy. Over time managing your condition becomes second nature and worry and fear drop off as you become more confident with your self-management.

Everyone will go through these stages of coping at their own pace and recognizing the various feelings and thoughts as you go through different stages is important as this is all part of the coping process. To help get through the coping process remember these tips.

Accept any feelings and thoughts you may have. There are many emotions you may go through during the coping stage and it is important to just let them come and go without giving them too much thought. Letting your feelings out by talking with someone can also be beneficial.

Ask questions and play an active role in your self-care by making sure that you know everything about your illness that you possibly can. The unknown can be frightening but if you know what you are up against you can deal with it much better. Learn what you can do to help your condition and what to do during the times when it seems worse.

Talk about your condition with others. Remember family members or loved ones will probably be going through similar feelings as yourself because of the empathy they may be feeling. Talk with family members and loved ones about your condition, don't leave them out of the loop

Keep things in perspective. When first diagnosed it can be easy to let your illness take over your life and let it become the most important thing. The best thing you can do is to keep things in perspective and carry on living your life just as you did before.

Understanding Asthma

Asthma is a condition that affects the small tubes which carry air in and out of the lungs. Irritants usually trigger an asthma attack and the effect of these irritants can vary from person to person. During an attack the muscles around the airways become increasingly narrower and the lining swells. Sticky mucus can also build up in the airways which cause further narrowing resulting in difficulty breathing.

There are a variety of reasons why you may develop asthma, but there are certain factors that can predetermine if you are susceptible to developing asthma such as:

Having a family history of asthma or allergies

Environmental factors such as changes in temperature

Smoking during pregnancy increases the risk of your child developing asthma

If you smoke you are more likely to develop asthma

Environmental pollution

Allergies to pets

The onset of asthma can develop after a viral infection

Irritants found within the workplace

The most common signs and symptoms of asthma will vary from person to person with some people experiencing some of the symptoms all the time while others only from time to time. Symptoms may include:

Coughing uncontrollably

Developing a wheeze due to the restriction of the airways

A shortness of breath

A tightness around the chest area

Asthma cannot be cured but it can be treated and kept under control very successfully. There are many types of medication that can help to successfully keep your asthma under control. These medications are divided into different categories which, depending on the severity of your asthma, you might have to use more than one of them. The categories include

Inhalers that prevent asthma

Inhalers that relieve asthma

Steroid tablets

Spacers

Nebulizers

Complementary therapies

Anyone who has asthma may have been prescribed an inhaler which is designed to quickly ease the symptoms of an asthma attack. The medication in the inhaler will help to open the airways making breathing much easier. It is important that if you have been prescribed an inhaler then you always make sure you have it near you.

If you have an infection and suffer from asthma then your doctor may give you a steroid treatment along with some antibiotics while you overcome the infection. A few people who suffer from asthma do occasionally need to take steroids long term.

Spacers and nebulizers are two ways that help you take your medication more easily. Spacers are usually given to children with asthma while nebulizers allow you to continually inhale medication through a mask which is particularly helpful during a bad asthma attack.

Living with Diabetes

Diabetes is a chronic disease that can increase the risk of developing other problems with your health. However there are many ways you can keep your diabetes under control and lead a relatively normal life. Living a healthy lifestyle, getting regular check-ups and managing your blood sugar levels successfully can go a long way towards successfully dealing with this condition.

Monitoring Your Blood Sugar Level

In order to control your diabetes successfully it is essential that you are able to monitor your own blood sugar level. There are a variety of home machines that you can buy which will give you accurate readings of your sugar level. Self-monitoring has the advantages of letting you be aware when your level is too low, will allow you to monitor your level during times of sickness and gives you confidence in the ability to successful keep your diabetes under control.

The best way to get accurate readings is to monitor your levels at different times during the day. There are small machines designed to be used in the home which very easy to use and include everything you need to stay on top of the disease and help you to control it.

Regular Check-ups

Getting regular medical check-ups is also a necessity. Check-ups are usually made every 3 months, 6 months or yearly and help to prevent complications from diabetes and ensures you are controlling it successfully between check-ups. During a check-up you will have your blood tested in order to monitor your glucose level. Your cholesterol level will also be checked along with having your blood pressure checked.

Other Risks

You may also be at risk of developing other illnesses along with your diabetes, such as heart disease and problems with your circulation so it is imperative that you look after your overall health.

Maintaining a healthy diet can go a long way to helping you keep your body healthy. You should remember to eat at regular intervals and include foods low in fat while high in fiber content. It is very important that you watch the amount of sugar you eat in your diet and also restrict the amount of salt you use in cooking and on your food.

Developing an exercise routine is also good for your condition, not only will it help to keep your blood sugar level stable, but will also help you to maintain a healthy weight.

If you have diabetes then you shouldn't smoke or drink alcohol. Smoking increases the risk of developing many other illnesses. If you do drink then keep it to a minimum and never drink alcohol on an empty stomach as this could lead to hypoglycemia.

Carpel Tunnel Syndrome

The bones and other tissues in your wrist help to protect your median nerve and together they form a narrow tunnel that is known as the carpel tunnel. Your median nerve is what gives you feeling in your fingers but occasionally ligaments and tendons get swollen and become painful as they press against the median nerve. When this happens your hand hurts or even becomes numb and you develop an extremely painful condition known as carpel tunnel syndrome.

Carpel tunnel syndrome most commonly affects people who do the same movements with their hands continuously such as clicking a computer mouse 8 hours a day. Those who are more at risk include typists, carpenters, grocery packers and assembly line workers, people with hobbies such as gardening, needlework, golfing and canoeing are also more at risk of developing carpel tunnel syndrome. It has also been linked with such illnesses as diabetes, arthritis and thyroid disease and women in the last few months of pregnancy can also develop it.

The first indications that you might be suffering from carpel tunnel syndrome include:

> Tingling or numbness in your hands and fingers, especially around the index, middle fingers and thumb.
>
> Pain in the palm of your hand, forearm, or wrist
>
> The pain or numbness is worse at night than it is during the day
>
> The pain gets worse the more you use your hands
>
> You have trouble gripping things and find that you drop them more often
>
> Your thumb feels particularly weak

Your doctor can perform an examination of your hand, fingers and wrist to help determine whether you have carpal tunnel syndrome. The examination may also include a nerve conduction test to help determine the diagnosis.

If carpal tunnel syndrome is diagnosed, treatment will usually consist of having to wear a splint which gives your wrist a rest. The splint can help to alleviate the pain particularly at night. Massaging the area of pain and putting ice on it can also help as can performing stretching exercises. In more extreme cases, surgery may also be a possibility. This is a condition that will improve with treatment but there are also some things you can do to help prevent the onset of carpel tunnel syndrome:

> Increasing your awareness of how you use your hands and equipment throughout the day can make a change

> Centering your work directly in front of you with your forearms parallel to the floor or slightly lowered

> If you stand up to work then have your workbench at waist height

> Make sure your hands and wrists are in line with your forearms

> If you work long hours at a keyboard then titling it can help

> Use proper hand and wrist movements when using a mouse and trackball

> Make sure you hold your elbows in close to your sides

> Make sure that you take a break every 20 minutes

> Do some stretching or flexing exercises every 20 minutes

Living with Arthritis

While arthritis is usually considered to be a condition that affects the older generations, it can also affect people of any age. It can affect any part of the body and there are thought to be over 200 different forms of this disease. However the three most common types of arthritis are osteoarthritis, rheumatoid arthritis and juvenile arthritis.

People who are affected by arthritis can go through many different emotions ranging from anger, frustration, worries for the future and concern about dependency. For the younger person affected by the disease feelings such as how other people will see them is a main concern. While the disease can be debilitating and make it difficult to be positive about the outlook, people do come to terms with this condition. Some of the ways that help to come to terms with the disease are:

> Talk about your feelings and fears. Getting your feelings out in the open is essential to coping with your illness. Talking with someone can relieve the feeling of anxiety and stress you may be feeling about your condition and how others may see you. Your confidant can be your doctor, a friend or family member or someone that is suffering from arthritis themselves.

> Learn how to relax and de-stress. Many people who suffer from arthritis get stressed easily and are unable to relax. You should learn routines that allow you to relax quickly and easily or find an activity or hobby that you could take part in to ease and forget about your stress.

> Seek help from a professional. If you don't feel you can talk to a family member or friend then seek help from a professional. This could be a counselor, doctor, social worker or a group in your area that deals with similar situations.

One of the most debilitating aspects of arthritis is the persistent pain it brings to the sufferer. However sufferers do seem to manage to keep the pain under control to a level where it doesn't interfere too much with their day to day life.

Here are some ways to help you deal with and manage the pain associated with arthritis:

Keep a note of the best time to take medication in order to get the best benefit

Notice when cold, heat and getting rest helps the most

See which form of exercise works best for you and when to do it

Keep practicing relaxation techniques

Take a pain management course

Purchase a device such as the TENS unit to help manage your pain

Consider hypnosis or acupuncture treatment

Attend pain clinics recommended by your doctor.

These are just some of the ways that people have been known to successfully manage their arthritis. Of course you should discuss with your doctor specific ways that could help you. Your doctor will also be able to advise you of any clinics in your area that you can attend to learn how to deal more effectively with this disease and the pain that it brings.

The Fear of Alzheimer's

There is no one single cause of Alzheimer's disease. Alzheimer's is brought on by varying factors with each person being affected differently. However, the biggest two factors which increase the risk of developing Alzheimer's are the advancement of age and heredity. Your degree of mental fitness and your environment are also thought to play a part to some extent although this and several other theories have not yet been proven.

Who gets Alzheimer's?

By the time you reach age 65, roughly 5 in 100 people have developed Alzheimer's to some degree. By age 80 the odds have jumped to 1 in 5 and almost half of all people at the age of 90 have some degree of dementia.

Alzheimer's isn't strictly limited to those over the age of 65, much younger people have also been affected by it. It is a disease that is thought to occur in women more than men but the main reason for this is simply that women tend to live longer than men.

Alzheimer's and Your Genes

There has proven to be a heredity link to Alzheimer's in roughly 3% of all cases of the disease. Heredity is thought to be the cause when the onset of the disease has occurred at an early age. About 40% of people who developed the disease before the age of 65 have family members affected by this disease. Just because you may have a family member with Alzheimer's doesn't mean you will be affected by it too. Quite the contrary. Although those with affected family members are at a slightly higher risk than others, there are still measures that can be taken to help avoid the onset of Alzheimer's.

Keeping Alzheimer's at Bay

Many believe that the environment in which you live can make a difference as to whether or not you are more susceptible to developing Alzheimer's. Research is currently being conducted as to whether exposure to certain metals is a contributing factor to developing the disease. Many experts have tied aluminum as a possible cause of the disease and suggest that antiperspirant deodorants should be avoided due to their high aluminum content.

Many doctors also believe that one's state of mental health plays a large part in the onset of the disease. The sharper one keeps oneself mentally the less susceptible one is to the disease. However there is not currently any evidence to suggest that staying mentally fit will make a difference one way or the other.

There are thought to be many other factors that could lead to the onset of Alzheimer's but additional research is needed due to the amount data. Some of the contributing factors include head trauma, various viral infections, a history of downs syndrome in the family, smoking and thyroid disease.

Alzheimer's and Your Future

Unfortunately there is currently no particular test that doctors can use to indicate who may be more susceptible to developing Alzheimer's. The primary goal in research right now is to better understand the causes and effects of the disease with the hope of one day being able to predict which people would be more susceptible to Alzheimer's before the disease actually sets in. By doing so scientists and doctors believe that it could lead to the development of treatments that could delay the onset of Alzheimer's.

Coping with Allergies

It is possible to develop an allergy to almost anything whether a smell, food, medication or reactions to dander found on animals. An allergy can range from nothing more than an annoying itch to the more serious effect of going into shock after developing a severe reaction. Allergies are usually divided into different categories that include:

Eczema and Urticaria which are allergies which affect the skin and include allergic skin rashes such as nettle rash and hives.

Hay fever which is a condition that causes reactions such as runny nose, sneezing, coughing and sore eyes during the summer months.

Venom allergies are reactions to stinging insects and snakes.

Adverse food reactions which people can be allergic to many different types of food.

Allergy to drugs whereby certain medications can cause a reaction in people. The usual reactions to drugs include a rash, sickness and stomach problems.

Anaphylaxis which is a severe and sudden intense allergic reaction that affects the whole body.

Asthma is an allergic reaction that commonly affects the breathing.

Eye allergies can vary from very mild irritation to severe conjunctivitis.

Are you Allergic?

If your doctor believes that you may have an allergy then steps will need to be taken to identify what allergen is causing it. The most common way of finding the allergen is to perform a skin prick test. The skin prick test is quick and relatively painless and the results are known immediately.

A small needle is used to gently prick your skin, usually on the forearm, with various allergens. The results will determine what allergens you are allergic to if your skin becomes red, sore and itchy around the area the needle was inserted. It is also usual for the area to come up in a welt. If you don't have a reaction to the allergen after a period of roughly 20 minutes then you aren't allergic to that particular allergen.

If it is suspected that you have dermatitis, which is a form of eczema, then you will normally be given a skin patch test. This test relies on taping patches with various allergens underneath aluminum discs. The discs are usually kept in place for a period of 48 hours and then assessed by a dermatologist for allergic changes.

Is it Severe?

In severe cases of allergy you might be required to have a challenge test to be performed in a hospital. The suspected allergens are then introduced directly into the lungs or nose and the allergic reaction is measured. If it is suspected that you might be allergic to food or foods then a double blind placebo test may be used. The food or foods that are thought to cause the reaction are given in a capsule under supervision while you wait to see if you develop a reaction to it. This type of test however is only done in extreme circumstances because despite it being the most reliable way it is also the most time consuming.

Acne Issues

One of the most dreaded 4-letter words for some people is acne because it often calls to mind dreaded terms like zits, pimples, whiteheads, blackheads, blemishes, clogged pores and unsightly skin. However dreaded doesn't have to mean hopeless because there is hope.

The main causes of acne are known and often easily treatable. For example, blemishes often appear because of body chemistry changes during teen years, menstrual cycles and menopause. Other factors are frequently due to too much bacteria clogging the pores and over scrubbing of the face in an attempt to get rid of the acne.

Treatments include over the counter anti-acne creams or solutions, prescription drugs and natural remedies. Some popular actions to take right away at home are:

Get an exfoliating cleanser and some anti-acne soap from the local drugstore or supermarket and wash your face gently with them every day. For best results wash as soon as you get up in the morning and right before you go to bed at night. And do not squeeze the pimples.

Get an anti-acne facial mask at the drugstore or find a honey facial mask which contains disinfecting and healing qualities. Use the mask up to two times a week.

Check with your healthcare provider about adding a multivitamin to your daily routine and a chromium supplement.

Keep hair back and away from your face especially your forehead.

Drink plenty of liquids daily, eight glasses of water is recommended. Eat foods rich in beta-carotene and vitamin A, like carrots, to help with skin repair.

Avoid putting makeup, paints, etc. on your face unless they are water soluble or marked as non-comedogenic and even then go very light on their use. And use a fresh, clean pillow case every day.

If you go out in the sun apply sunscreen with SPF 15. Whenever possible choose one that's also non-comedogenic or non-acnegenic so that it doesn't clog your pores. Add a hat and sunglasses and skip those tanning beds.

Common Misconceptions about Acne

When attempting to rid yourself of acne, it is best to know what works and what is well intended folklore. Here are some of the more common rumors surrounding acne treatments:

Greasy foods, stress and chocolates can cause and increase acne problems. This is a myth. There is no scientific evidence that supports this.

Squeezing your pimples can help get rid of them. This is also untrue. Squeezing can actually make matters worse forcing infection further below the skin's surface and can even cause scarring.

Being out in the sun can help dry up acne. This also untrue. Too much sun can actually make things worse by drying out your skin and causing irritation not to mention wrinkles and increasing the risk of skin cancer later in life.

Controlling Your Blood Pressure

You should have your blood pressure tested at least every 2 years because high blood pressure can lead to such problems as damaged blood vessels among other things. High blood pressure can increase your risk of heart disease, heart attack, developing kidney failure and stroke. Having your blood pressure checked takes only a few minutes and should there be a problem your doctor can treat it and recommend changes to your lifestyle that you should follow. Here are some simple tips to making changes in your lifestyle to keep your blood pressure within a normal range.

Smoking is a No No

If you smoke then you should definitely quit. When you inhale the smoke from cigarettes and other tobacco products, your blood vessels become restricted which causes you to have a faster heartbeat. When your heart beats faster this causes a temporary rise in your blood pressure. By giving up smoking you not only help to lower your blood pressure but you also reduce the risk of heart disease and heart attack.

Your Weight

Losing weight and getting enough exercise can help towards keeping your blood pressure down. If you are carrying too much weight around, your heart will have to work harder and faster and this can cause your blood pressure to rise which increases your chances of developing heart disease and stroke.

Alcohol in Moderation

Limiting the amount of alcohol you drink is also important. In some people alcohol raises their blood pressure significantly while in others it doesn't seem to have as much effect. You should drink no more than 1 glass of wine per day or one can of beer and if your blood pressure does rise through drinking, then you should quit drinking altogether.

Avoid Excessive Sodium

Some people can be affected by sodium which in turn causes their blood pressure to rise. If you have been diagnosed with high blood pressure then it is important to reduce the amount of sodium in your diet. You should not add extra salt to your food and always check food labels for the levels of sodium contained in foods.

Decreasing your Level of Stress

If you live a very stressful life and easily become stressed then this can cause your blood pressure to rise. It is important to learn ways of dealing with stress and not let it build up. There are many self-help techniques that you can learn to help you combat stress such as meditation, deep breathing exercises, yoga and visualization.

Treating High Blood Pressure

If your doctor has diagnosed you as having high blood pressure then changes in your lifestyle are necessary. Your doctor may also prescribe medication as an effective way of controlling your blood pressure. There are many different types of medication used in the treatment of high blood pressure. In some cases if your condition can only be controlled by medication, then it could mean that you have to take medication for the rest of your life to help keep your blood pressure under control. However the earlier you start making changes to your lifestyle and begin leading a healthier life, the better your chances that you won't need to be on medication for life.

Chapter 5

Natural or Alternative Healing Methods

The Basics of Alternative Medicine

Alternative medicine is a term that refers to medical practices outside of conventional western practices. Alternative solutions are sometimes new and untested in the scientific realm of conventional medicine. They sometimes focus around or contain a religious, spiritual or metaphysical element. Here are some popular alternative medicinal solutions.

Apitherapy

Better known as bee therapy, is a practice that makes use of honey and venom from the honeybee for treatments. Raw honey, bee pollen, royal jelly and propolis are some of the more popular ingredients used for health and beauty products and healing treatments.

Biofeedback

Refers to a technique you can use to learn to control your body's functions, such as your heart rate. The feedback helps you focus on making subtle changes in your body which healthcare providers chart to help with treatment. These techniques can more accurately chart internal functions than a human alone is capable of and the results are used to determine and then gauge how well the treatment is working. Biofeedback has been used to help people with emotional disorders, digestive disorders, stress, migraines and heart irregularities. This technique also alerts people to the idea of how their own emotions and thoughts can come into play with regards to illness and treatment options.

Chiropractic Services

A form of treatment that focuses on the vertebrae not being aligned properly thus contributing to a variety of pain, illnesses and diseases. Some chiropractors also focus on stress, overall health and lifestyle. In general a chiropractor applies pressure in small amounts to various vertebrae helping them to realign. Additionally many also help treat common diseases such as asthma, troubled backs, and arthritis.

Feng Shui

Is a philosophy that is said to bring harmony into a person's life. It features not only the four basic elements of earth, fire, water and air but a fifth element; metal. By aligning these elements throughout clutter-free homes, work, outdoor and other environments; peace and tranquility are said to follow.

Healing Crystals

These are minerals turned crystalline that are said to boast certain healing powers. For example ancient grave sites house them as a means of protection in the afterlife. In the modern world many believe these crystals contain healing powers that can cure various illnesses such as stomach pain just by placing a charged quartz on the lower abdomen area which helps to restore energy there.

Herbal Remedies

These can be either home grown or store bought herbs that when applied to certain ailments helps to heal those ailments. Among popular treatments are a half-and-half solution of witch

43

hazel and water to help clear up acne, lavender scented oils and candles to sooth stress and garlic on top of warts to remove them.

There are many more alternative medicine treatments for various conditions and an internet search for alternative medicine will reveal a plethora of information.

Chinese Medicine, a Holistic Therapy

Chinese medicine is a complete holistic system that can lead to a healthier, happier and more stress free way of living. It is a system that people have benefited from for over twenty-three centuries and is used to diagnose, treat and prevent a wide variety of illnesses and problems.

The different aspects that make up Chinese medicine all basically rely on the same principle, Yin and Yang, which represent the two opposite principles in nature. Yin characterizes the feminine or negative nature of things and yang stands for the masculine or positive side. Yin and yang are pairs, such as the moon and the sun, female and male, Light and dark, cold and hot, passive and active. The basis behind this is to restore harmony and peace to the mind and body which the Chinese believe can eliminate many diseases and illnesses.

Qi is the life force that flows uninterrupted throughout the body and is similar to blood throwing throughout the veins. It is when there is a disruption in this Qi that problems and illness occurs. Restoring the flow of the Qi restores harmony and dissolves the symptoms of illness.

The two main components of Chinese medicine are acupuncture and herbal remedies.

Acupuncture

The art of inserting tiny needles underneath the skin that stimulate targeted areas of the body. Acupuncture is most often used to relieve pain and heal the body. Acupuncture focuses on the Qi that flows throughout the body through points known as meridian points. While it is flowing freely we are healthy and happy, but if the channels become blocked then the Qi stagnates and this leads to symptoms of various illnesses depending on where the Qi is blocked. Acupuncture works when the practitioner restores the normal flow of the Qi by stimulating the meridian points of the body.

Herbal Treatments

Chinese herbal medicine is usually dispensed after an acupuncture treatment although it can be used as a standalone treatment. There are over a thousand common herbs that are used in various combinations for numerous problems and illnesses. But there are two main types of herbal remedies that are commonly used in treatments. These are "food herbs" and are generally eaten as part of the diet and are mainly used for prevention of disease and illness and maintenance. "Medicinal herbs" which are usually prescribed by a doctor of Chinese medicine and are specially prepared for the patient based on the individual's needs. The formula is made up from the patient's medical condition, the environment and the constitution of the person being treated. Medicinal herbs are usually given along with acupuncture treatments which aids in the "re-balancing" of an individual's life force.

The benefits of Chinese medicine are numerous and has been thought to have helped many physical conditions along with increasing mental clarity. Here are just a few of the conditions acupuncture has been known to treat successfully.

Sinusitis, bronchitis and asthma

Conjunctivitis and cataracts

Stroke, sciatica and osteoarthritis

Faster recovery from injury

Improved circulation

Relief from stress and anxiety

Relief from pain

Strengthening of the immune system

Addictions, phobias and eating disorders

Aromatherapy

Aromatherapy, a term created in 1920, involves the use of essential oils that are compounds in their purest state. The oils are concentrated liquids derived from plants through a variety of means including distillation, solvent extraction or expression processing. The resulting oils are then used as treatment for a variety of ailments and healing.

Aromatherapy was actually coined because of Mr. Rene-Maurice Gattefosse. My Gattefosse was conducting research about how oils might aid in healing, when his arm caught on fire. In an attempt to put out the fire he accidentally poured lavender oil onto it which caused the arm to heal faster leaving no scar. Since that time many practitioners have used aromatherapy and essential oils to help with physical and emotional healing.

Common Uses of Aromatherapy

Some common uses for aromatherapy oils are as scents for homes and offices which help trigger relaxing feelings from occupants and to also help get rid of unwanted smells and germs. For example, lighting candles and burning wax chips made with aromatherapy oils can help rid a kitchen of smelly fried onion and other food smells.

A light fragrance can help welcome people home after a long day at the office. Popular scents are bergamot, eucalyptus, lavender, jasmine and rose.

Some of the oils, like lavender oil, can help fight bacteria. And others, camphor and menthol for instance, can help increase your metabolism and endocrine system, improve your central nervous system and boost your immune system to fight colds.

Other aromatherapy oils are also used during massage treatments. Absorbed by the skin and muscles, the oils activate thermal receptors that result in warm relaxing feelings and calmness in the muscle groups.

And still other aromatherapy oils when applied to the skin are used as topical aids which aid in the destruction of microbes and other fungi. Some oils are taken internally where they can help improve antiseptic activity, stimulate the immune system and work as a diuretic.

Cautionary Use of Aromatherapy

When deciding about the uses of aromatherapy for your ailments and healing, use the following guidelines as precautionary measures:

Pure essential aromatherapy oils can be very strong and harmful to animals, children and yourself, so check labels carefully before using aromatherapy products and consult your healthcare provider if needed. Do not use in pure undiluted oils on your skin.

Do not use aromatherapy oils if you are pregnant or have epilepsy or asthma.

Test the ingredients and sample a drop or two first to check for any allergic reactions.

Only use aromatherapy oils in small amounts as they can cause burning of the eyes or have other negative reactions.

Let Go of Depression Without Drugs

On the face of it trying to get rid of depression without using drugs seems to be hopeless, especially these days when most people have gotten used to the idea of being treated with prescriptions drugs. But many people are successfully turning away from prescription drugs and finding alternative methods of treatment without drugs. Those suffering from depression are finding cures through therapy without drugs which do not cause any side effects and are typically much more economical.

Blue Lights

Depending upon the cause of your depression, you will need to choose an appropriate type of therapy. If your depressive disorder manifests itself in winter when days are short and daylight is sparse, you may effectively make use of phototherapy. Bright light therapy or blue light therapy is given with the help of a light box which reduces or removes the cause of this type of depression.

Counseling

Psychotherapy can be helpful in cases in which psychological factors are identified to have caused depression. In such cases psychotherapy or counseling will work better if there is good understanding and a solid rapport between the counselor and the patient. Depending on the severity of the disorder long and frequent counseling sessions may be necessary. Thought patterns, personal relationships, and low self-esteem are some of the issues to be identified and corrected. Self-loathing has to be converted onto self-love and stress has to be lowered or eliminated and so on. During these type of sessions the most important thing is the approach the counselor brings to the table as well as the relationship between the practitioner and the patient.

Exercise

Physical exercise is also considered to be a very good cure for depression particularly when it is combined with psychotherapy. It is an effective method of ridding excessive stress that may be causing the depression. Although it may be difficult to encourage severely depressed people to try to be physically active, persistent efforts aimed at motivating them to get involved in regular physical activities may be necessary for the benefit of the patient. In practice group physical activities are known to alleviate depression by addressing the root causes of the depression.

Foods and Supplements

In certain cases of depression dietary supplements like those which are rich in Omega-3 fatty acids (particularly those found naturally in oily fish) can work as a remedy. Products containing chocolate and Vitamin B-12 are proven to also be effective as antidepressants along with some herbal substances. When depression occurs due to misuse of alcohol and other intoxicants, such as caffeine, sleep-inducing drugs and sedatives, the obvious remedy lies in abstinence of these depression triggers.

Meditation and Spirituality

Meditation and deep breathing exercises are being increasingly used as a means of treating depression without drugs. These have produced results proven to be very effective especially when practiced regularly. The calming effect of meditation on the mind has a positive impact for depression sufferers as does prayer and spirituality.

Rehabilitation of depressed people is a family and social responsibility. Often times a depressed person is just looking for the attention of loved ones and in these cases attempts to treat depression by drugs alone will not be successful. For this reason the stigma that is associated with mental illness, like depression, has to be discarded. Loved ones must provide support and not treat the depressed person like a leper because this can make the situation even worse. Love and support is the best way to begin remedying depression.

Get Enough Sleep

Most of us don't realize the true value that sleep can have on our bodies and minds and the majority of us don't get enough of it. For some of us this could be due a sleep disorder such as insomnia, while for others just staying up too late and getting up too early can cause sleep deprivation. Getting enough quality sleep is not only essential to help us get through our day but also for our overall health.

Not getting enough quality sleep can have adverse effects on our bodies and consequently adversely affect our health. When we don't get enough sleep our body begins to crave more carbohydrates and sugar causing our blood sugar levels to fluctuate. Not getting enough sleep can also cause problems with our adrenal glands. The adrenal glands regulate our body's health and when our adrenal glands start suffering our body is adversely affected.

Another problem in not getting enough sleep is an increase in the hormone cortisol. Elevated levels of cortisol interfere with learning and memory, lower our immune function and bone density and can cause increases in weight, blood pressure, cholesterol and heart disease. Cortisol levels are supposed to drop at night time allowing our bodies to relax and recharge. But if our cortisol levels are too high, we might notice that even if we've been tired all day, we get a second wind right around bedtime.

So what can we do to ensure that we get enough sleep? Here are some tips that may help:

Avoid eating before going to bed and if possible do not eat after 7pm. The later you eat the less time your body has to digest food before going to bed. Instead of resting the body will spend all night digesting the food that was eaten. Also going to bed on a full stomach will lead to feeling uncomfortable and subsequently tossing and turning all night.

Get enough exercise throughout the day to help your body become tired thereby making sleep come easier. Regular exercise not only gets you fitter but also helps you to get a good night's rest.

Dim the lights at night because just as the sun streaming through your window first thing in the morning starts your day off by energizing you; dimming the lights at night can encourage your body to slow down and unwind.

If you are having trouble getting comfortable in bed at night then consider buying a new mattress. If your mattress is old and worn this could be the reason you are tossing and turning all night.

Develop a healthy internal clock by getting yourself into a routine. Get up at the same time every morning and go to bed at the same time every night.

Whenever possible stay awake during the day and don't take a nap. Taking a nap during the day confuses your internal clock and you are not as tired when it comes time to go to bed.

Avoid turning your bedroom into an office. Don't put a desk or your computer in there and avoid the temptation to work. If you have work in there you are more than likely going to be thinking of the things you have done or should have done and this can keep you awake.

Try winding down with a hot drink, hot chocolate or warm milk, before going to bed but avoid coffee or tea as they contain caffeine which can keep you awake. Of course give this enough time to go through your body before lying down for the night otherwise you may wake up in the middle of the night with an urgent need to go to the bathroom.

Conclusion

This book is not all inclusive as there are many ways to help you on your journey to a better, healthier lifestyle. However by using this as a starting point you can be well on your way to a much more fulfilling and longer life. Keep in mind to check with your doctor before starting any exercise regimen or a radical change in your eating habits.

For many of us implementing any of these suggestions for healthy living may be very difficult. Taking the time to research what to eat, the proper vitamin intakes, being sure to drink enough water and finding the exercise routine that will get us moving may seem daunting at first. Add to that the reality that we must find the time to get enough sleep. In order to live a long and healthy life we must make a commitment to start healthy habits as part of our daily routine.

Finally, we should always listen to what our bodies are telling us when we are sick or feel "out of sorts." This is the body's way of telling us to recognize that we aren't leading as healthy a lifestyle as we should. If we make some of the simple changes mentioned above we will go a long way towards getting our mind and bodies back in shape.

The world is filled with various lifestyles so make your life your own by staying healthy and avoid sweating the small stuff. Making sound decisions is a great start to live a long and healthy life.

www.ingramcontent.com/pod-product-compliance
Lightning Source LLC
Chambersburg PA
CBHW062020280526
45787CB00005B/2182